My Son
Through
My Eyes

MY SON
THROUGH
MY EYES

Based On A True Story

Sally McGuire

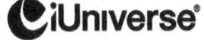

MY SON THROUGH MY EYES
BASED ON A TRUE STORY

iUniverse books may be ordered through booksellers or by contacting:

iUniverse
1663 Liberty Drive
Bloomington, IN 47403
www.iuniverse.com
1-800-Authors (1-800-288-4677)

ISBN: 978-1-5320-7558-2 (sc)
ISBN: 978-1-5320-7559-9 (e)

Print information available on the last page.

iUniverse rev. date: 05/20/2019

Dedication

In loving memory of Jordan.

The heart never forgets. You will never be forgotten

Authors Note

To me, a hero is an ordinary human being who finds strength to persevere and endure in spite of overwhelming obstacles. When I was seventeen, I was standing in a room at a friend's house and saw a picture, taped on a wooden partition, of a beautiful woman. She had the most attractive smile. The photo was one of the few happy things in a house weighed down by poverty.

'Who is this woman in this picture?' I asked smiling with admiration in my eyes. I thought that she was the most beautiful woman that I have ever seen.

As the years went by I saw how she took care of her love ones. Even though she lived in another country, nothing prevented her from taking care of her responsibilities. They look to her for everything and she never disappointed them. She would call; write letters, send money and packages with things that they need. I recall one time when one of the packages that she sent to them accidentally went all the way to Africa. That did not discourage her from sending more – she continued doing so diligently. I would ask about her regularly because I was very impressed by her love, commitment, kindness and generosity. She reminded me of myself on so many different levels even though she was old enough to be my mother.

Four years later I migrated to the United States and by some miracle fourteen years later I reconnected with her eldest son. I got the opportunity to talk to her for the first time when her son was battling an incurable disease. I witness her strength, her weaknesses and the great love that she had for her child. I was amazed by her faith and strength as she fought for him.

As time gone by, she has proven to be a great source of strength for me as well. I appreciate her words of wisdom and her advice. 'Always be the best you Sal,' she tells me. 'Never let people's actions or words stop you from doing so.' She tells me to always protect my heart, stay hopeful, and be mindful that this world is filled with horrible people who will inflect pain on others for no reason. I care about her even though we have never met. I have the most love, admiration, and respect for this amazing person.

This woman is my hero. One of the most rewarding things that I have done as an author is writing this book. Thank you for trusting me with this special piece of your heart. Destiny has brought us together and I will always be grateful.

Sally McGuire

My wonderful son,

You are one in a million and I love you.

God gave me a gift in you.

Love Mom.

"Being a mother

Is learning about strength you don't know you had,

And dealing with fears you never knew existed."– Linder Wooten.

Introduction

Motherhood to me is the most important job in the world. It is not a job where you are rewarded with a salary or promotion for a job well done. To carry a child for nine months, listen to its heartbeat for the first time, feel it move, and to finally give birth is truly miraculous. Watching your child grow, teaching him or her about life—love, hate and right from wrong—can be extremely challenging yet most rewarding. The love in their eyes when they look to you for guidance, protection, or comfort is priceless.

To be a mother is a role that I take very seriously. There is no instruction manual stating what I should or should not do. I made mistakes along the way, but I hope that they did not affect my children in any adverse way. I used these errors as learning experiences to help me to do better as I dealt with my grandchildren and great-grandchildren. The love and pride that I felt in my heart as my children grew and matured into successful men and women was the greatest reward ever.

My dream or wish as a mother was always to see my children living happy, meaningful, fulfilling lives, to see their dreams become realities: getting married and having families of their own. I could never imagine living a life without my children. I would not be the kind of woman that I am today. They taught me patience, unconditional love and so much more. They made me want to be a better person. My experiences in the process made me stronger and wiser.

I gave my children advice, but I never told them how to live their lives or made decisions for them. Sometimes they messed up by doing things that were not beneficial for their overall happiness. They did not always seek my advice, and often I had to stand by and watch them make their own mistakes. It was not always easy, and sometimes it broke my heart. I would simply pray and let them know I was there if they needed me, always.

Seeing their child sick and suffering is the most heart-wrenching thing for a parent. When they cry, the parent cries, too. No good parent stands by helplessly watching their child's future being ripped away from them by illness. Instead, they do everything in their power to prevent it. The worst thing that can happen to a parent is to hold their sick child in their arms as they draw their last breath. I am a mother and my son died of cancer at the age of twenty-seven. This is my life story.

Chapter 1

I was born on a tropical island in the Caribbean. The island was colonized in the 1600's and was later controlled by Great Britain in 1967. For many years, slaves cultivated sugarcane and produced molasses and liquor, which were sent to Europe. In 1974, the island became an independent country; however, the Queen's presence is still represented today. When I was growing up over fifty years ago, agriculture was the main part of the economy. The island produced a wide variety of spices such as nutmeg and cinnamon, which were exported to other countries. Jobs were scarce and the economy grew at a slow pace. Many families lived in poverty. Some had to fight for everything—including an education. A few privileged ones had a good standard of living on the island, but for most life were hard and hopeless. When I was young, the only thing that kept me going was my hopes and dreams for an amazing future. I was the eldest of four children and like most first-born was given a lot of responsibilities. I had to do house chores, work the land, and help take care of my siblings. I loved to play with them.

On the island, there wasn't much for young boys and girls to look forward to as they grew older. If you were fortunate enough to attend high school, you would probably end up being a teacher, or getting a job at one of the local banks. Life was extremely hard for my family: it was a struggle just to get the basic necessities. My father did his best to provide and take care of us. He and I had a very close relationship and he always made me feel like a princess. I remember him taking me for walks, going hunting, and doing lots of other fun things. We would talk for hours even though I was very young. We talked about my hopes and aspirations, right and wrong, and so much more. He wanted me to attend high school when I got older and even made preparations for me to do so. He called me "Queen" and every day he showed me how much I was loved—he was my hero and I loved him very much.

My father was murdered when I was thirteen years old and things became much harder. I felt as though I had lost a piece of my heart. He was the one person who loved me unconditionally and now he was gone. I had to take on most of his responsibilities and help care for my love ones since my mother was ill. I cooked cleaned, hand-washed laundry, prepared meals and so much more. I did this for years as my childhood was taken away from me. While most teenagers were dating or hanging out having fun, I was busy taking care of the people I loved. I did not have much time to attend school, but the few times that I did, I took advantage of it. Life was very hard for me: I had no one I could trust.

I had lots of relatives on both my parent's side, but I came to the realization that most did not have my best interests at heart. Some made sexual advances towards me so I avoided them and learned to depend on myself. The world became a dark place and I was unhappy. I worked odd jobs like working in a store that printed t-shirts. I had no choice. I wanted to be a normal teenager, but I could not without putting my love ones at risk. At times I felt alone and misunderstood. I cried sometimes as I mourned for my father and the loss of his love—especially when faced with challenging or difficult situations. I dreamt of a better life where I was happy and could also be stronger for those who depended on me.

My social life was non-existent, though I had many admirers. A few of the boys and girls in the village would speak to me when I passed by. At eighteen, I met a young man and we became friends. He wanted a future with me, but I had my doubts and eventually ended it. At twenty, I became pregnant—not an unusual thing in my culture, for a man whom I was friends with. Most girls had kids when they were teenagers. I desperately needed to find stable employment in order to provide for my Child and continue helping my love ones. Things were getting worse and I needed to find ways to make them better. Jobs were difficult to find in the rural part of the country where I lived, and the few that were available were ones for which I was not qualified. I did not have many skills or qualifications since I did not finish high school. The only skill that I had was typing—I had a typewriter someone had given to me.

I traveled to the city to seek employment and was fortunate enough to get a job as a cook at a restaurant. I moved to the city, which was convenient since it was very expensive to commute to and from work daily. It was a long distance from home and bus fares were high.

I thrived at my job because cooking was something that I was good at. I met people from different walks of life and cultures and the experience helped me grow mentally and socially. I was not home every day and I missed my baby. I paid bus drivers who worked on routes close to where my family lived to deliver groceries, money, and other things as they needed them. They would drop it off at a local gas station and a family member would pick it up. I was constantly worried about them. Did they have enough to eat? What did my newborn child need? Would I be able to provide it? I did all that I could to make their lives better and neglected myself and my own happiness in the process.

I did not have many friends, nor did I have much free time. Although I tried very hard and things improved somewhat—it still was not enough. I lived in poverty and there were people who looked to me to make their lives better. I also wanted more for my child and for myself. I wanted to be happy, have peace of mind while at the same time providing basic necessities for those I loved: a nice home, for instance.

I kept dreaming of a better life where I was happy and accomplishing all my goals. I wanted my love ones to live prosperous lives and lack nothing. When the opportunity came for me to travel to the United States, it seemed like a dream come true. I was promised a job and the chance to help everyone who depended on me as well as myself.

Though the proposal seemed promising, I was skeptical. The idea of traveling to a faraway country with a stranger was intimidating. I was pressured by my mother whom I trusted, however, into believing that it was my only choice if I wanted to make a better life for the people that I love. Reluctantly, I agreed and accepted my fate.

I was told that the United States was a place where all my dreams would come true, that it was a place where I would be happy. I envisioned working and going to school, making lots of money and helping my love ones and eventually moving out on my own, with my child. These ideas were great motivators and at the naïve age of twenty-one I arrived in the United States leaving behind my young son. I had no idea how drastically my life would change.

At first, United States was fascinating: sprawling mansions, wide boulevards, different ethnicities and varied cultures. Growing up in a third-world country, all of this was both alien and intriguing: I was eager to start my life in this amazing place. I had everything planned out in my mind and I was filled with anticipation.

My excitement soon turned into misery: I was forced into marriage with the man who had given me the opportunity to come to the States. I was not in love with him. He had been a friend of my mother and I was barely acquainted with him. So I found myself married to a stranger, far from my home, away from everyone I loved.

My situation rapidly deteriorated into abuse. I was never allowed to go anywhere alone. My husband accompanied me everywhere. Most of the time I was home alone, cooking and doing housework. My sole purpose was to facilitate his happiness and I was a prisoner in my own home. I became depressed and lonely, with no idea how to get out of my situation. I thought of my love ones, especially my young child, and I prayed to God for help.

Though I was going through a terrible time, I remained strong. There was no room for weakness or failure, and I found other ways to cope and persevere. The hardships of my youth had prepared me for the challenges I faced in my marriage. My husband assured me that money was being sent to my family on a regular basis, and that gave me some small peace. I would go shopping with him and purchase items that we later shipped to my country. I wrote letters to my love ones and there was the occasional phone call when one of my relative could go to a neighbor's house and use their phone. I was always anxious to hear about my child. They sent me a few pictures of him, and I dreamed of holding him in my arms once more. I was promised, if I was an obedient wife, that someday he would be brought to the United States to be with us. I held onto this hope as years went by.

My husband wanted to have a lot of children—ten, to be precise. I did not want any more children, given my situation. After my son was born, a friend and I had gone to a local clinic where I elected to get an IUD by a doctor. My husband had no idea and after five years of trying to get me pregnant he became angry and took me to an OB/GYN to find out why it was not happening. The doctor informed him as to why I was not conceiving. My husband became furious and I was accused of deceiving him. I was given medication, to make me more fertile. Still, I did not conceive. I was verbally abused, called degrading names which in turn made me more depressed. I was made to believe that something was wrong with me. Once, when we were out walking, I smiled at a woman with her baby. "That is a real woman," I was told by my husband. Those words hurt me deeply and there were moments when I became physically ill and my body seemed to shut down. I saw a doctor who gave me medication that provided only temporary relief. All the while, I cooked, cleaned, did laundry and tried to be a dutiful wife. Soon enough, I became pregnant.

When I found out I had conceived, I was happy and relieved. I would no longer have to deal with my partner's abuse. I was also comforted by the fact that I would soon have someone to love me and I would not be alone anymore. My husband worked most of the time and was rarely home.

I had been leaving In the United States for the past five years and I was totally dependent on my partner. I had no friends, no bank account, no library card, and no social life. I had a difficult pregnancy and was frequently ill. Still, I persevered, taking care of all my husband needs: he never let me forget my obligation to him.

On one of my prenatal visits I discovered we were having twins. I was ecstatic! Two babies! Sadly, during the first trimester I lost one baby and I was at risk of losing the other. My doctor placed me on bed rest, telling me I was working too hard. I rested as much as possible, taking vitamins and trying to eat right. I gained a lot of weight, but I did not mind. I prayed a lot as I bonded with the child inside me. I would talk to him and sing to him. He was my hope for the future, and I felt comforted every time I felt him move inside of me.

On September 30th, 1986, after eight hours of labor, I gave birth to my six pound, eight ounce son. His strong cry was music to my ears. I gazed at his full head of hair and admired his perfection as I fell in love. I named him, after my favorite basketball player, but called him Buddy because that what he was to me – my Buddy.

As the months went by, I watched Buddy grow and blossom. I was amazed by everything that he did. He was an energetic baby—so full of life. I witnessed his first smile, first time sitting up and every other milestone that babies go through. Just to look at him brought immense joy and happiness to my heart. I was still dealing with some medical issues which were very painful and challenging. Taking care of a young baby, being a wife and caring for a family were very difficult, but my son gave me the strength and motivation to go on.

My doctor diagnosed me with cervical cancer, which was very distressing. I had seen a doctor regularly and I could not understand why I had not been diagnosed earlier. I had been treated multiple times for infections, so the cancer was a shock. I watched shows about cervical cancer and what it could lead to and I was frightened.

I did radiation treatments even as I still cared for my baby and took care of all my other responsibilities. My little boy gave me the will to survive. I looked in his big brown eyes and all I felt was love. I would read to him and feed him and know that he was the most fulfilling thing in my life. Buddy would be strangely calm when he drank his formula. He also liked to be soothed by riding in a car. My husband would drive us around at night and I would take my son with me on the local bus. I felt alive and free when I was allowed to take the bus for the first time. I would visit shops, parks, and restaurants. I marveled that I had lived in the United States for over five years and knew nothing about the community in which I resided. I looked forward to my outings on the bus.

It was on one of those bus rides that I met and made my first friend. She lived in the apartment complex where I lived and sometimes we would ride the bus together and talk about our lives. Life was much better for me now. I had my son who was healthy and growing well and a friend to talk to. I was happy to share with her some of the things I was going through. I had kept all of my struggles to myself, which was not healthy. She was very kind and sympathetic. I would tell my friend about the island of my birth, my first born child, and my family and how much I missed them all. And, I would tell her about my husband.

She was baffled when I spoke about my controlling spouse and the mistreatment I endured. She was also my age and she educated me about my community and how things were done. She advised me on the importance of having my own bank account and other things that would help me gain independence.

Buddy and I had a very close bond. He was a loving child, always giving hugs and kisses. I took him with me everywhere. People always told me what a handsome baby he was. He had big brown eyes and a mop of thick black curls that grew thicker as he got older. He was also full of energy and started walking at ten months. On days when I was sad, tired, or just sick I would hold him in my arms and that gave me the strength to keep fighting. I never talked baby-talk to him, but spoke to him like an adult. He was a blessing to me in a difficult time.

Childhood injuries, bumps, scratches, or boo-boos are not unusual, but when it happened to my son for the first time it was one of the most frightening moments of my life.

He was about a year old and I had put him to sleep on my bed. I was in the next room watching television. Every so often I would look in on him, making sure he was ok and sleeping peacefully. On one of these occasions, I noticed blood on his pillow. I could not determine where the blood was coming from. I immediately called my husband, who rushed us to the hospital. We later found out he had an infected tooth, which he had gotten from sucking his pacifier.

My child was a happy, energetic toddler and sometimes I was amazed by how much energy he had. As I gained more independence from my husband, I started venturing more places on my own and doing things by myself. Life became less depressing as my son and I did things together. We would go to the supermarket, where he loved to ride in the cart. He assisted me when we went to do the laundry. I smiled when he would attempt to fold clothes or put them in the laundry bag. He always wanted to help me with my chores. We would go to the park and play for hours without getting tired or bored. His favorite toys were cars. Whenever we would go to a toy store, he would always wander over to where the cars were.

One day, we were outside when a modeling agent approached me. He was impressed by how handsome my son looks and thought he could be a successful child model. I was very excited when we did a photo shoot for the modeling agency. Buddy looked so handsome dressed in his red shirt and red and black sweater. I was so proud. Later, I was informed by the agent that I had to be available at any time to take my son to auditions or travel all over the US. I realized that was not the life I wanted for him. I wanted him to go to school and be with children his age, so I pulled out of the agency.

My son started school at the age of five and we were both very excited. I can vividly remember his first day of school. Thinking about it always brings a smile to my face. He got up very early in the morning and began dressing himself in his white shirt, blue pants, blue jacket, and white socks and shoes that I had laid out for him. When he was finished dressing, he took his small backpack and placed it on his back, smiling up at me. "I am so proud of you, Buddy," I said. I was so delighted at his independence. He looked so handsome in his school uniform and was eager to begin his first day.

I, however, was a bit apprehensive and somewhat scared. I did not know how he would adjust to a classroom environment. We had never been separated and he had not socialized much with children his age. Knowing I had to leave him at the school did nothing to allay my fears. When we got to the school, I met his teacher, and she gave me a tour of his classroom. I greeted other parents and observed the setting. I began to feel confident that this was the right place for my child. After lingering for a little while, I started to exit the room. "Don't leave, Mommy!' Buddy cried, holding onto me tightly. I tried to comfort him and reassure him that I would be back to get him soon. My heart was breaking as I pulled away. The image of his pleading brown eyes haunted me for the rest of the day until I returned the school to pick him up. We were both extremely happy to see one another. This pattern continued for a few days until he finally acclimated to the routine.

Starting school was not an easy adjustment for my son. He was very "hyper" and had difficulties in settling down, which created lots of problems with his academic growth and development. He was not able to read like most kids his age. It was very frustrating for me, because I knew how intelligent he was. He would have articulate conversations with me and figure out things that most five-year-olds did not do. I knew that he was quite capable of reading well. I had an obligation to see to my son's education and I did not solely depend on his teachers to teach him to read.

My son loved going to the park, and that is where I taught him to read. After I let him run around, climb trees and play with other kids for a while we would sit down with a book. It took a while and I had to be patient as well as persistent, but in time we made progress. *Clifford the Big Red Dog* was the first book he read by himself. He was very proud, and I was even prouder.

Chapter 2

There were lots of changes in my life by the time my son started first grade. I was now a single parent with four kids. My husband had left, and I had to care and provide for my children. He was three years old when I had my first daughter and a year later, I had another. I also had a financial obligation to my oldest child and family in my homeland. I needed to find a job in order to take care of all my responsibilities. It was not easy and very frustrated, but I had to find a way.

I noticed that there was a demand for child care service in my neighborhood and surrounding area. I saw lots of kids in the park when I would take my children to play there and learned that there were not many day care centers in the area. I researched what it would take to start a child care service in my home and then got all the necessary licenses and certifications. I also took in foster children, becoming a foster mother. The job was perfect for me because I loved children and I was able to care for my own children at the same time I was working.

I worked very hard for long hours to be successful at my job. I had many things to learn, but I was determined and did not consider failure as an option. The mere thought of not succeeding only motivated me further. Lots of people, including the children as well as the parents, were depending on me and I could not let them down. After a while, my hard work paid off and my day care was considered to be one of the best in the area. I had lots of children and my foster children were also thriving.

My own children thrived as well. We all had a great relationship and I encouraged them to work together as a family unit, even when they were young. They were expected to help with small chores in and around the house. We worked as a team and I was proud of them. I was continuing my treatment for cervical cancer, which was a tedious process. At times it was hard for me to focus on my health with all of my responsibilities. I did whatever the doctors recommended, took my treatments and prayed that all would be well. I also made a friend who was a great help to me and my family. I was thankful when my health changed for the better and the cancerous cells in my cervix were gone.

I was now an independent, working woman with a home, bank account, credit cards and so forth. I did not own a car because I did not have a driver's license, but I hoped to accomplish this at some point in the future.

From the second grade forward, school was complicated for my Buddy. He was constantly disrupting his classroom by jumping on tables, throwing things all over the room and engaging in other negative behaviors. He also had difficulties following directions and could not sit still.

The school phoned me frequently, complaining about his behavior. Sometimes the teachers asked my permission for him to stay after school and clean up his messes as a form of discipline. I would speak to my son about his behavior and punished him as often as I could, but nothing seemed to work. It was frustrating for me and I often lost patience and yelled at him. It was as though he had no understanding of the consequences for his actions.

At home, he could be loving and kind but was still full of energy. He climbed on everything, including the refrigerator door. He was always jumping around like a wild animal. He loved to play with the foster children and his younger sisters, but he was sometimes a bit mischievous. I recall one day where he cut off his sister's braid and thought it was funny. My son was still helpful to me, helping to care for the smaller children in daycare and doing chores around the house. There was never a dull moment with my son.

I routinely took my children to the library—at least once a week or more if I could. I knew the importance of their having an appreciation for reading at an early age. A thirst for knowledge would be a great asset for their futures. My two daughters loved books and would read a wide variety. While they were busy reading, Buddy's main interests were in pictures or videos of cars. One of the few books that he loved to read was Beatrix Potter's *The Tale of Peter Rabbit*. He loved Peter Rabbit and thought he was the coolest rabbit ever. I bought him a stuffed Peter Rabbit, since I knew how much he loved the character. He was incredibly happy and would sleep with it on his bed.

Most of all, my son loved cars—all kinds of cars. That was basically the only toy he wanted to play with since the time he was very small. I would bring him to the toy store and he would head straight for the toy cars: he wanted to be a race car driver. I remember when his father asked him what he wanted to be when he grew up, and that was his answer. His father told him forcefully that he needed to be a doctor or an engineer and not a race car driver. Race car drivers did not have steady incomes nor make enough money, according to his father.

"You can be anything that you want to be, Buddy," I said when I saw the sadness in his eyes. I wanted him to know that his future was bright. He smiled back at me and I knew he believed everything I said.

In time, my son was diagnosed with Attention Deficit Hyperactivity Disorder and dyslexia. ADHD is a common behavioral disorder that impacts focus, self-control, and other skills important in daily life. It is caused by differences in brain anatomy and wiring and often runs in families. The disorder affects about 10% of school age children. Kids with this diagnosis are hyper-active, act without thinking, and have a hard time focusing. The diagnosis made me understand why he behaved the way he did and why he did not understand the consequences of his actions. I became more patient and tried to figure out ways to help him. I also better understood his reading disability. Kids with dyslexia have trouble learning and interpreting words, letters and other symbols. I knew Buddy was nonetheless intelligent: he was always inquisitive and asked many questions.

My son was very kind-hearted and caring. The only time I remembered him being hurtful or violent to anyone was one time when he hit his classmate. His teacher called me and asked me to come to school. When I got there and the teacher told me what my son had done, I was shocked. I asked him why he had hit his classmate, but he would say little in front of the teacher. Later, he admitted that the kid was making fun of the spots on my skin. I had a condition called Vitiligo, which caused patches of my skin to become white. He was protective of me and did not like his classmate saying mean things about his mother.

I was always concerned that my son would hurt himself because he was so hyperactive. I kept my eyes on him constantly. One day when he was nine years old, he got badly hurt. He was playing outside and wanted to ride his bicycle. I told him that he could, but to be very careful. I knew he was not responsible enough to ride his bike without supervision, and I told him I would be watching him. He began to ride his bike up and down in front of our house.

I watched him for a few minutes and he was doing great. Then, not surprisingly, he began to ride his bike faster and faster. "Buddy! Slow down!" I screamed as he rode past me with a big smile on his face. He ignored my warning and peddled even faster. In the blink of an eye, he was thrown from the bike: he flew through the air and landed on the ground.

"Oh my God!" I screamed as I ran to him, my heart racing. "Buddy! Are you ok?"

"Mommy!" he cried. "My leg hurts!"

I could tell he was in a lot of pain. "You will be ok, Buddy," I told him.

His leg was badly injured, and I called 9-1-1. An ambulance came and rushed us to the hospital. When they x-rayed his leg, the doctors told me it was not broken but was severely bruised with injuries that could cause permanent damage if he did not receive immediate treatment. He had to be given injections, and I had always hated needles. My son noticed when I looked away as they administered the shot. He began to tell me that needles were nothing to be afraid of. He told me that he was not scared, and he was right: he didn't even flinch.

My son had an ability to make me do things that were out of my comfort zone. One day we were hiking near Palm Springs. There were many scenic overlooks and the children were excited to look out from the viewing decks. Everyone was having a marvelous time except me: I was terrified of heights. Buddy looked at me and said "Mommy, don't worry. Nothing is going to happen to you. Hold my hand."

I looked in his eyes and saw the faith that he had in me, and in turn I believed everything he said. My son had an amazing way of allaying my fears and making me more self-confident. After that day, I was never afraid of heights again.

My Son doctors informed me that medication was the best treatment for his ADHD. I did my research on the condition and disagreed strongly; I did not want my child to be dependent on medication at such a young age and I refused to give it to him. I believed that there were other things that could be done to help him and other kids with the disorder. For example, attending special classes with different activities that would help channel their energy and keep them active. I strongly believed that medication should be the last resort. There were lots of people who disagreed with my decision. My son's school had a huge problem with my choice because he was destructive in his classroom and struggled in his studies. They thought that my decision endangered my son and called in Children's Services. Children Services began to be at my house constantly. Their incessant questions and observations were irritating. They also spoke with the school about his conduct. They even investigated his bike accident, as if they were trying to prove that I was an unfit mother. Nothing came of their investigations, but they did not go away and the school still pressured me. I was forced to make a heart-breaking decision: my son would go to the Caribbean and live with my relatives.

I was told that Buddy would have lots of space to run and play and that he would get to know his older brother. After he arrived in my native land, I soon received confirmation that I had done the right thing. My family informed me that he was doing great. He ran to and from school each day in the tropical weather. He was doing well in his studies and making friends. There were many outdoor activities like playing ball, climbing trees or flying kites. He loved animals, so his relative presented him with a black sheep. Buddy named her "Black Beauty" after the story I had read to him. He cared for her, fed her grass, and spoke to her like she was a person.

I was also informed that my son was loving and kind—something I already knew. He bonded with his older brother and offered hugs to his love ones. He always said "Please" and "Thank you".

I missed my son very much and I continued to send money and care packages and whatever else he needed. I knew I had done the right thing for him, but it did not make things less painful. I thought about him every day. Sometimes I felt like I had abandoned him in his time of need.

Before he went away, my Buddy gave me a present: a picture of two pigs sitting on a bench. One was bigger than the other and wore a pink scarf. The smaller pig wore a blue scarf. They were hugging one another and smiling.

"That's you and me, Mom," I remember him saying. His big brown eyes were full of love and adoration.

A year went by and I couldn't be parted from my "buddy" any longer. I made all the necessary arrangements to bring him home. I counted the days and stocked up on all his favorite foods and other things he loved. When he finally arrived, I was amazed at how much he had grown. The sun had darkened his skin and he had a healthy glow. His sister and I could not hug him enough. I looked in his eyes and I knew he had missed me as well. A piece of my heart had returned, and I vowed I would never send him away again. Whatever problems came our way, we would handle it as a family.

Chapter 3

Raising children is not an uncomplicated job, yet it's incredibly fulfilling. There are always challenging and frustrating moments that arise, but one must always focus on doing what is best for the child. My kids meant everything to me, and I did my best to make sure they had quality lives. I watched them grow and develop into individuals, each with their own talents and traits.

There were times when I was not proud of the way I spoke to them or the way I meted out discipline. I only did what I thought was best or what I knew. I had never had anyone set examples for me as to how to be a good parent. I did not have the best role models, so I read books and watched television shows on how to be a better parent and tried hard not to repeat the blunders that I had experience or seen committed. Still, at times I found myself doing just that. Though I tried my best, at times I simply messed up. During those occasions, I evaluated my actions and vowed to do better next time. I only wanted my children to have good foundations and solid futures—the things I had never had.

I loved being with my children and doing different activities with them. We celebrated birthdays, Christmas, went skating and did lots of other fun things as a family. I settled disputes between them, comforted them when they were sad and tried to do all the things that loving parents should do. I was both father and mother and strived to give them normal, happy lives. They were my top priority and there was not a day that went by that I did not show them how much I loved them.

When my son came home from my homeland, he was much calmer and went back to school initially with little incident. I was delighted with his progress and hoped that his good behavior would continue. Soon, he fell back into his roguish ways. Although his conduct was less than stellar, he continued to excel academically. His grades were above average when he graduated elementary school and entered high school.

When I think about Buddy as a teenager, I beam with pride. He was tall and handsome and still had his thick, black curls. He had an eye for fashion and loved dressing in designer clothes. Timberland and Nautica were his two favorite brands. He always looked as if he had just stepped out of a fashion magazine. Red was his favorite color and, like me, he loved the Chicago Bulls. He couldn't resist pasta and was fascinated with cars and the outdoors. He was also very shy and would never be the first one to reach out to a stranger or initiate a conversation. He had few friends and was quite particular in his tastes and habits. He always cleaned his shoes after he wore them and would put them away neatly. When he went shopping, he examined merchandise carefully. If there was the slightest imperfection, such as a dropped stitch, he would not purchase the item. Though there were many positive changes in his life as he matured, he still continued to misbehave in high school. –

Most of my son's mischief-making was to make others laugh. His actions never hurt anyone, and for that I was thankful. One day, he broke into the football team's locker room and stole all their sport drinks. He then handed them out to the kids in his class. He and the others thought it was funny, but the principal, teachers and coaches did not. I was immediately called to school—something I had grown accustomed to. Whenever the phone rang during the day, my first thought was, *what has my son done this time?*

I was told that I could either pay for the drinks or my son could help the janitor clean up after school. When I spoke to him about his actions, he dismissed me and acted as if it were a big joke. His attitude angered me and I elected to make him assist the janitor as his punishment.

There were many instances when I was incredibly frustrated with my son's behavior and did not know how to reach him. I would have done anything just to make him change his troublesome ways. I had spoken to him, yelled at him and even punished him over the years but nothing seemed to work. He was constantly in trouble. I never gave up on him, though, and I tried to make him understand that his behavior was unacceptable and that there would always be repercussions. I worried constantly for his future and hoped and prayed that he would calm down. I feared that my Buddy would do something that might get him expelled from school or placed in juvenile detention.

The bond between Buddy and me became stronger as he got older and we dealt with all his problems together. I told him on many occasions that he could talk to me about anything: and we did. I did not care how horrible things got—he needed to know that he could come to me. I would always be there for him, even in the most difficult of times. I knew that my son was misjudged and misunderstood because of his actions. He needed to know there was one person who would not judge him. When he did something that I did not approve of, we would talk about it. He would help me at home or in the daycare without any complaints. He did chores like cleaning the bathroom and taking out the garbage. He also helped feed the children.

My son had a wonderful relationship with his sisters, particularly his youngest. They would play and watch movies together for hours. I loved the bond they shared. He was one of the most kind and compassionate person I knew. I recall one occasion when he demonstrated what a caring heart he had.

One afternoon, after school, my son walked into the house with two homeless boys. They had been part of the foster care system, but were now living on the streets. He wanted me to provide them a place to stay. I could see that he genuinely felt sorry for them and I had to break a few rules when filing the necessary paperwork for them to come live with us. It was the right thing to do, and his sympathy for the two boys was my primary motivator. The boys became his best friends.

As Buddy grew older, he continued to push me out of my comfort zone. I never thought I could learn to use a computer and kept all my daycare records manually. He encouraged me to learn to use a computer, telling me that I needed to keep up with technology. I made all my usual excuses, but he would hear none of them and began to patiently teach me to use a computer.

Many girls were interested in my son, but he was very shy. They fawned over his thick curls and the way he dressed. They came over to visit frequently, as most of his friends did. He never strayed far from home.

One late night, around one in the morning, I heard voices coming from Buddy's room. *Who was in my son's room so late at night?* I rushed to the door and barged in to find him seated on his bed with three girls. I began to curse and immediately phoned the girls' parents, asking them if they knew where their daughters were. After his company left, I continued to argue with him. "What was going on in your room, Buddy? Do you have any idea how disappointed I am in you? You should know better!"

My son flashed me his smile. "Relax, Mom. Those girls are just my friends. We were only hanging out watching a movie."

"Are you sure that was all you were doing?" I asked.

I looked my son straight in the eyes as I could always tell when he was lying. He reassured me that they were only friends and I believed him. Slowly, I began to calm down. My son had his whole future ahead of him and I didn't want him doing something stupid. I knew he was going to have girlfriends, but I didn't want him to be a teenage father. I told him that having children when you are too young changes your life forever. I knew all too well. I also didn't want him to contract any STDs and I encouraged him to be safe and make wise choices.

I'll never forget the time that my son came to me and informed me of his first date. It had been a busy day in the day care and I was rushing around. He came up to me and started conversing with me as I managed the children. He seemed to be in an exceptionally good mood, and I asked him why. "I have to escort a girl to her Sweet Sixteen birthday party," he replied with his shy smile. I was mildly surprised. He was not the sort of boy who would ask a girl for her telephone number, much less for a date. He would always stand on the sidelines and wait for a girl to come to him. "How did this come about, Buddy?" I asked him.

He explained that the girl's mother had approached him and had asked him to escort her daughter. He had asked the woman why she chose him, and she had replied that she was impressed with how handsome, well-dressed and polite he was. "That's wonderful," I told him. "Are you excited?" He told me that he was, and that the daughter was "cute".

We immediately began preparing for his big night. He got his hair cut and picked out a new outfit. On the night of the dance, I was incredibly proud of my son. He looked so handsome in his suit, tie, and dress shoes. He was very happy, although he was also a bit nervous. The next morning, I could not wait to ask him how his evening went. He told me that he and the young lady had a wonderful time and had decided to start dating. I was happy for him as she was a nice girl. They fell in love and became high school sweethearts.

My son was not "sweet" on high school, however. He was branded as a troublemaker and I was constantly trying to make him understand how critical his education was. I provided incentives and rewards whenever he got good grades. I promised him new sneakers, clothes, and whatever else he liked. One day, I said to him "Buddy, I'm going to buy you a car." He was wide-eyed. "Really, Mom?" I replied that I was serious and that I would buy him a car *only* if he graduated from high school. Knowing how much he loved cars, I figured this would be good incentive for him to get his diploma. I was right.

My son graduated from High School in 2004. I was so happy and proud that he had reached this point of his academic journey. I was a little disappointed when he told me that he did not want to wear his cap and gown and march with his class at the graduation ceremony. I respected his decision, however. His high school experience had not been the most pleasant and he just wanted it to be over. Now, with a diploma, he could at least go to college and build his future. I told him that he had his whole life ahead of him and that there was nothing he could not accomplish if he persevered.

I also kept my word and bought Him a car: a Buick Regal. He was overjoyed as he inspected the car inside and out. I'll never forget his smile as he took it for a spin around the neighborhood.

Chapter 4

Communication plays a huge role in life and is essential for any relationship to grow. It was extremely important for me to keep the lines of communication open with my children for my family to be happy. They needed to voice their opinions and talk about whatever was going on in their lives. After my father died, I had no one to talk to about my life, my fears, and my hopes. Mostly, I was made to believe that I had no right to be heard or give my opinions. I was told what I should or should not do without any consideration of how I felt or what I really wanted. This was damaging to my personal growth and development. I ended up withdrawn and had low self-esteem. I thought that no one cared about me. I did not want any of my children to feel the way I had felt.

Over the years, I would take the children to Malibu Canyon where we would have our "family meetings". The surroundings were beautiful and there was a feeling of freedom. I gave them the opportunity to express themselves in whatever way they desired. They would talk about their issues and frustrations and we would discuss ways to deal with them. By communicating with my children, it helped me to see where I might be going wrong. Those moments were special for all of us.

After Buddy graduated from high school, he decided to take some time off before starting college. I did not have any issues with his decision as he had assured me that he would start college the following year.

He spent the time doing things he loved: hiking, fishing, going to the beach and other activities. He developed an interest in firearms and began going to a shooting range. After obtaining his license, he began to purchase guns which he stored in a safe place.

I was amazed at how much calmer my son was at this time. He accepted responsibility and had control of his life. The only time he was reckless or aggressive was when he drove his car. He loved to drive fast and sometimes he raced other cars. He also bought and collected remote control cars and drones. Whenever they got damaged or mangled, he would go to the store and purchase the parts to repair them. He took good care of his car and had fun working on it and accessorizing it. Sometimes he would drive me on errands or we would just ride around. We would talk about many things as we rode along. I cherish the memories of those times. They reminded me of the days when he was little and it was just him and me.

"Mom," he asked me one day on a drive, "would you care if I drive fast?" I looked at the gleam in his eyes and then I looked out at the beautiful, sunny day. There were only a few cars on the streets. "It does not matter how fast you drive, Buddy," I told him. "I'm not scared." We both smiled as he raced along, enjoying the thrill of the moment.

There were other amazing things that my son and I did together—moments that I could never forget. Like the time he took me to the Redwood Forest in Los Angeles. I was amazed to see how tall and beautiful the trees were with their different colored leaves. We were able to do a little hiking and explore some of the natural beauty in the forest. He explained to me how the leaves changed color. He and I were in awe as we became one with nature.

I was now at a good place in my life and was happy and thankful, even for the simplest things. I kept on working hard and doing what I had to do for my life to be more productive. My daycare and foster care were functioning smoothly. Kids came and went, and I always had a feeling of accomplishment, knowing I had helped them grow and develop. My family was happy and complete since my first born was now with me. I also got married for the second time to a man who had been my devoted friend for many years.

Two years have gone by and still my son was not in college, nor did he have a job. I spoke to him constantly about his future and he often told me that I worried too much about it. I did not care, since I wanted only the best for his future. I tried and tried to convince him that he could not go on living his life this way, doing nothing. I had lived a life with no education, and it had not been easy. His life had to be different, so I gave him an ultimatum. He absolutely had to get a job.

It was about this same time that Buddy informed me that he and his girlfriend, who was living with us, were expecting a child. This was not the news I wanted to hear, though I wasn't exactly surprised. He and his girlfriend had been together for some time.

"Are you ready to be a father?" I asked him. "You are very young and being a father is a big responsibility." He replied that he was ready and that he had thought about being a father since he was very young. "Is that so?" I asked, quite shocked by his response.

"I know, Mom," he said. "I will be a good father."

We converse some more and I saw how happy and excited he was. We talked about things that needed to be done as he prepared for the role of a father. My children were not fortunate enough to grow up with a father in their lives. I believed that he truly understood the responsibilities that came with fatherhood. I was willing to give him the help and support he needed as he embarked on his new journey.

My son started his first job at a construction site a few months later. He was thrilled to work at a job where he would be doing the things that he loved. He drove machines like Bobcats and tractors and other heavy equipment. He could not wait to take me and his love ones on a tour of his job site. I saw how proud and passionate he was as he skillfully maneuvered the machines. In a few months, he got a promotion and the advance in salary was incentive for him to work harder. He was in a good place in his life.

My son and my relationship was a loving one most of the time. There were times, not surprisingly, when disagreements occurred. They became more frequent as he got older and wanted to do things his way. Some of those moments were intense and heart-wrenching. I vividly remember the day we had one such conflict. I had asked him to contribute money towards the household since he and his girlfriend were living with me. I was also still taking care of my relatives in my homeland at the time, as well as my own family. I thought it only fair that he now help with the bills and I asked him to pay one monthly bill. My son became indignant and refused. "Why should I pay any bill?" he asked.

I was baffled at his response as he expressed his displeasure in a most disrespectful manner. His words were hurtful and insulting as he told me exactly how he felt. I could not believe the things he was saying. Tears filled my eyes. *Who is this man speaking to me?* Was this my "buddy"? The young man standing before me with his big, angry brown eyes must surely be an impostor!

For days, I could not get the incident out of my mind. Every time I thought about it, I would cry. Sometimes I would ask myself where I went wrong as a parent. I taught my children right from wrong so that they would grow up to be respectful men and women, but it seemed as though I had failed them, based on my son's actions. I used that experience as a learning tool to help me deal with similar instances that occurred with him or any of my other children. In time, my son apologized. It took me some time to get over it, but I eventually forgave him.

I saw how thrilled and keyed up my son was as he prepared to be a father. He went with his girlfriend to her doctor's appointments, shopped for the baby and did all the things that newly expectant parents did. His son came early at seven months. He was there through the delivery, watching his son come into the world. After he was born, the baby was placed in ICU because he was still quite small.

My son visited the baby regularly. Those visits were difficult for him and his girlfriend. It was not easy for them to see their little baby hooked up to tubes and monitors, with nothing to do but hope that their child would soon come home with them.

Since the baby had come early, there had been no baby shower and there was plenty to do to get ready. We needed diapers, clothes, a crib, a car seat and so on. My son and his girlfriend had everything ready when the baby was discharged from the hospital. He had even bought an outfit for the baby to wear when he came home. I saw the love and excitement in his eyes as he took on the role of father. He was great at it, using much of the learning he had acquired in the day care. He got up in the night with the baby, fed him, changed his diapers and bathed him. I was very proud....

Nothing in life remains the same. Things change, sometimes for the good and sometimes not. This is life's reality. I watched the way that my son dealt with change over the next several months after his son's birth. He was laid off from his job that he loved and decided to go to college. He took courses at a local community college, majoring in accounting. He excelled in his studies and even talked about opening his own bank one day. In the meantime, his relationship with his girlfriend ended, and that made me very sad. My grandson was young and needed both his parents to raise him together. I had to raise my children without a father and I knew how difficult it was, especially for the children. It was hard to spend holidays and birthdays without a father. It was hard not to have a father at their school activities. I did the best I could, but I knew things would have been different had both parents been in my children's lives.

Reluctantly, I accepted my son's and his girlfriend's decision. He and the mother decided to co-parent amicably, though at times it wasn't easy. I was proud of the way he continued to be dedicated in his role as a father.

Buddy was happy, doing whatever he wanted to do as a young man. He made choices and decisions about his life— some of which I did not agree with but respected anyway. He excelled in college and had plans to transfer to his dream university in Southern California; the college he had always wanted to attend. One day, he showed me an essay that he was working on and it melted my heart as I read it. The speech prompt was to give a toast in a mini-tribute to a person for what they had done and to express a blessing for the future. He chose to write about *me!* He wrote how his mom had always stuck by him no matter what, and how I had encouraged him to go to college but had never pressured him. He thanked me for always loving him, even when he didn't deserve it. I was impressed by what he wrote, and though I knew he loved me, it was then that I realized just how much we meant to each other. The feeling was mutual.

My son dated, raced around in his car, explored the outdoors and continued to do the things he enjoyed. He was a wonderful big brother to his sisters, who looked to him for advice and encouragement. He had a great sense of humor and was never too busy for them. He was doing well, and his future looked promising.

One day, my son came to me and showed me a small lump on his leg. He was worried as he had noticed it in the shower and had noted that it had rapidly changed. I had looked at it before and assumed it was nothing serious and had told him not to worry. This day, however, the lump looked and felt different. I did not like what I saw and told him that we needed to make an appointment with a doctor. We went to our family doctor, who had been caring for me and my children since they were born. The doctor expressed concern and referred us to a specialist.

I was not worried when my son went to see the specialist days later. I believed that he was healthy and strong, since he had never had any major health issues before. On all his trips to the doctor, he was given a clean bill of health. I deem that it was just a routine checkup and the lump was nothing serious. The doctor would find out what caused it and take care of it.

When he came from the specialist that day, I could tell that something was wrong. He had fear in his big brown eyes as he looked at me.

"Buddy, what's wrong?" I asked.

"The doctor thinks I have cancer," he replied softly.

"What do you mean? Why would he think you have cancer?" I blustered. I could tell he was confused and in shock.

He explained that even though the lump looked small on the outside, it was huge on the inside. He needed to have surgery as soon as possible. I could not accept what he was telling me, and I began to cry. How was this possible? My son had cancer? This could not be true. There had to be another answer. I looked at him and saw his uneasiness. He needed me to be strong for him.

"Don't worry, Buddy," I said. "We will figure this out together." I hugged him tightly and reassured him that they would take the lump out and all would be well. I passed on my positive energy to my son and he believed me, as he always did.

On the day of the surgery, I went with my son. We were both nervous, but anxious to get the lump removed and find out what caused it in the first place. I reassured him once more that everything would be fine and I would be right by his side. The nurses did his blood work, vital signs, blood pressure and an x-ray. When it was time for my son to do the x-ray, I was present in the room with the technician. I wanted to see what was going on, even though I could not read the results or understand what was happening. I just wanted to be there for him.

I looked at the images and was baffled by what I saw: it did not look normal, even to a layperson like me. There were spots everywhere. My heart began to race and I asked the technician what the results were. He told me that the doctor would explain everything shortly. I was terrified. I knew something was wrong.

"Mom," Buddy asked me, "what did you see?"

I remained quiet since I did not know and did not want to scare him unnecessarily. We had always had a strong connection and he saw the worry in my eyes. He looked at me and I knew he wanted me to tell him the truth.

"Mom, just tell me," he said.

I told him that the x-ray was covered with spots, but tried to set his mind at rest by telling him that it may not be anything serious and everything was going to be fine. I did not want him to worry about anything. He listened to me and did not say much. I could tell that there were a million things running through his mind as he tried to process everything that was happening.

When it was time for the surgery, I was with him as far as the staff would allow me to go. I kissed his cheeks and forehead and I held his hands and prayed with him. He was scared though he was trying to be brave and strong. I reassured him once more that all would be well and that when he opened his eyes I would be right there. My heart broke into a million pieces as they wheeled my "Buddy" away.

Time dragged on as I waited for the surgery to be over. I walked at a slow, easy pace up and down the hospital lobby, praying for my son. I was nervous as a million thoughts raced through my mind. I refused to consider that anything bad would happen to my son. This would be a minor surgery and when it was over, he would be fine. I returned to the waiting room and watched as a woman and her child passed by. I had seen them earlier and I struck up a conversation. A few minutes later, a nurse entered and informed me that the doctor wanted to speak to me. I anxiously made my way to his office.

"Ma'am," he addressed me when I arrived, "I would like to talk to you about your son's condition. There are some things that you should know."

"What is wrong with my son, Doctor?" I asked abruptly.

"Ma'am, your son has cancer. It is very serious, and he is going to die."

"What?!"

"Your son has cancer, and it is very bad," he repeated.

I could not breathe—I felt like I had been punched in the gut. I struggled to process the doctor's words: *My son is sick and he is going to die?* My mind screamed, *No!* The doctor was wrong. It could not be true! I began a barrage of questions and was overwhelmed by the answers. *This could not be happening!*

I looked at the doctor as he continued explaining my son's diagnosis, and the reality of what he was saying finally hit me. I started to scream and tremble as tears fell from my eyes. I did not care where I was or who heard me. All I could think about was my son and what the doctor had just said. The thought of my Buddy not being a part of my life was something that I could never accept.

"Ma'am, you son is asking for you." I turned to see the nurse standing in the doorway. "He is waiting for you in the recovery room."

I suddenly became conscious as to where I was and quickly tried to compose myself. I needed to control my emotions and be strong for what I had to do next. My Buddy needed me, and I had to be there for him. I wiped the tears from my eyes and slowly followed the nurse to the recovery room, my heart breaking with every step.

When I got there, my son was lying on his bed. He was still hooked up to tubes and recovering from the anesthesia. He opened his eyes and looked at me as I walked towards him. He studied my face as I sat down next to him. My face was tear-stained and my eyes were red: he knew something was wrong.

"What did the doctor say?" he asked. "Just tell me, Mom."

I told him the doctor said that he had cancer and that it was bad. I looked at him as he remained quiet and emotionless. I could tell he was in shock and trying to process the information. My son was only twenty-three years old!

"Am I going to die?" he asked softly.

I took him into my arms. "I do not care what the doctor says. You are not going to die!"

My son felt so fragile in my arms. I wanted to protect him and keep him safe. I vowed to never leave his side until this nightmare was over. I would fight this battle with him, and we would win.

"Don't worry, Buddy. You are going to be fine. We will fight this together!"

Chapter 5

My son was diagnosed with Alveolar Soft Part Sarcoma. It is a rare type of cancer where soft tissue grows slowly. The cells of origin are unknown, and it occurs mainly in children and young adults. ASPS can migrate into different parts of the body, typically the lungs and brain. His cancer was Stage 4, and he was given six-to-twelve months to live.

I spoke to my children about their brother's diagnosis the day we came home from the hospital. It was a heart-wrenching moment for my entire family. They cried and pummeled me with a million questions. They demanded that I seek another specialist and get a second opinion. I comforted them, answering their questions to the best of my ability. It was by far the worst crisis my family had ever faced.

"'Don't worry. Your brother is going to be fine," I told them, trying to be strong for my children. My son looked frightened and my other kids were confused and worried. They did not know what to believe.

Soon afterward, I asked the doctor who diagnosed my son for a referral to a different specialist. He sent me to doctors in my area. They too concluded that my son had Stage 4 cancer. They were nonetheless optimistic and were willing to work hard to help him. They did not know much about this form of cancer, but they believed he had a fighting chance. I observed my boy as the specialist spoke: he was listening attentively. They sent us to an oncologist to begin treatment.

When we arrived at the clinic, I was very disappointed. The building was depressing and stark: no paint, no flowers. The atmosphere was far from welcoming. The staff was unprofessional and most of the patients were elderly people who seemed to simply be waiting to die. I concluded that this was not the place for my son. I spoke with the oncologist there and he told me about a clinic in the Santa Monica area that specialized in my son's form of cancer. We promptly made an appointment.

The clinic was everything that I hoped it would be. My son was very excited as we toured the area. The treatment center was modern and equipped with experts, friendly staff, state-of-the-art diagnostic tools, laboratories and so much more. What I loved most about the place was its loving and welcoming atmosphere. The staff was friendly and there were patients around my son's age. These patients had access to television, video games and other things to keep them as happy and comfortable as possible. He was relieved that we had found a place to facilitate his battle with a horrible disease.

I began right away to obtain all the necessary documents needed for Buddy to start his treatment with, a sarcoma oncology specialist at the Santa Monica clinic. I gathered his medical records, referrals and other documents the facility required. I could not wait for the insurance company to process his claim. For the next few weeks I checked my mail daily, anxiously awaiting a letter.

My upbeat attitude was soon shaken when my son's insurance rejected our request to pay for his treatment. I was extremely upset and could not understand why. The insurance stated that they would only cover treatment at the former facility. They indicated that the clinic had the same qualified doctors and protocols. I related the news to my son and he was instantly devastated: he had his heart set on going to the clinic in the Santa Monica area. I knew, still, that the former clinic was not the place for my son.

He looked at me with his soulful brown eyes. "Mom," he said, "If I don't go to Santa Monica for treatment, I won't beat this cancer."

"Don't worry son," I said. "I will take care of everything. You are going to the clinic in Santa Monica for your treatment—I promise."

Over the next few weeks I made numerous calls to the insurance company, to doctors, clinics, and anyone else I thought could help me. I made numerous calls to the insurance company, doctors, and clinics—to anyone who I thought might help me. I put all the numbers and the dates and times that I called in a folder, just to keep track of what I was doing. This process was frustrating as I wasn't getting any positive results. Sometimes I got very upset and, feeling powerless, I would break down and cry. I prayed a lot though, and I never lost faith. I kept reminding myself of my son's faith in me. I had to make this happen. Time was running out and he needed help *now*. I continued to fight with the insurance company and they continued to reject my request that he go to Santa Monica.

"Why can't they just help us?" I screamed one day.

I began to think of other ways to get money for my son's treatment as I battled the insurance company. I had little savings and I could not refinance my home…I needed a miracle.

One day, I called the insurance company yet again. A woman answered with a soft and courteous voice. After we exchanged pleasantries, I told her that I needed someone to listen to me.

"Do you have children?" I asked her.

"Yes, I have three kids," she replied. 'Yes, I have three kids,' she replied softly.

"I need a guardian angel right now," I said. "I need you to help me."

I then told the woman about my son's diagnosis and how the insurance company was not willing to pay for him to be treated in a special clinic. I made it clear that the clinic covered by the insurance company was not going to do much to help him. I pleaded with her desperately, telling her that the Santa Monica clinic was the place that could save my son's life.

"I will help you," the woman said after she heard my story. She explained that she had a senior position with the company.

She gave me instructions on what I needed to do next. I first had to get a signed letter from the oncologist, stating that he could not treat my son at his clinic. Afterwards, I would fax the letter directly to her as soon as possible.

My heart beat with anticipation as I hung up the phone. My miracle was on its way. I immediately made an appointment to see the oncologist. When I got there,

I explained the situation, which was delicate as it was disingenuous for him to write a letter stating that he could not treat my son, when in fact he could. He understood my desperation and agreed to write the letter. We decided that he would continue as my son's primary doctor while he got his treatment in Santa Monica. He and a doctor from Santa Monica would work together as a team to give my Buddy the best care possible. I was over the moon as the oncologist signed off on the letter.

"I admire your strength and perseverance as you fight for the welfare of your son," he said as he handed me the letter. "You are right: this place is not the best place for your son's treatment." He went on to say that he believed my son had a fighting chance by going to the clinic of our choice.

I thanked him for everything, including his honesty, and I left. Now, things were finally going to happen. My Buddy would get his treatment and he would beat this cancer.

I faxed the letter directly to the lady as she instructed me to do. The insurance company approved the treatment and sent me a confirmation letter. I was overjoyed! I had prayed for a guardian angel and God had sent her to me. I also shared the good news with our family doctor, who was amazed by everything that had happened. He said that it was indeed a miracle that the insurance company had approved the treatment. He wished my son the best.

My son began his treatment almost immediately. He took chemotherapy for two weeks and then had a two-week break. He would come home every day after chemo, instead of remaining at the clinic, bringing along a machine that had to be attached to his body.

I will never forget the time when my Buddy had his first round of chemo. The oncologist talked to us about the drugs and the side effects. Fatigue, nausea, vomiting, hair loss, reproductive issues were all things that might occur. When he and I got home that day, he immediately got in his car and drove off. I was concerned that he was by himself and had just taken a treatment. My concern grew into panic as the hours went by and he had still not returned. I contacted friends and family to find out if they had seen or heard from him. I feared that he had been involved in an accident and I could not sleep. When he finally came home, I rushed to him in relief.

"Buddy! Where have you been?" I asked. "Are you ok?"

"Mom, I am fine," he replied. "I went to the Malibu Canyon- a quiet place I love. I just wanted to think."

"I was so worried about you," I said with a sigh of relief. It was totally understandable that he needed some space after dealing with his treatment and the doctor's prognosis. So much was happening to him in his young life. I was happy that he was coping in his own way, though I reminded him not to worry me like that again.

My son will drive himself to and from his appointments with me by his side. We were very optimistic that the treatment would work. I was astonished by his strength, since he was experiencing some of the side effects of the chemo and yet still largely participating in his usual routine. He spent hours educating himself about his illness, always searching out new treatments and discussing them with the family. I was astonished by how intelligent he was.

There were many changes that took place after my son started his first round of chemo. His thick mop of black curls that I loved so much began to fall away. He did not let it bother him. He immediately shaved off all his hair as he looked at me and smiled. He was handling the changes to his body with bravery and acceptance. He rarely complained about anything. As the treatment continued, he began to lose his appetite and started losing weight. He grew weak and I began to tempt him with all his favorite foods: waffles, pasta, tangerines, grapes, and so forth. Every night I made his favorite Café Vienna. Then I would massage his back, legs, face and feet. We would talk about everything except the cancer. He would try to talk about his treatment, but I would immediately change the subject. I refused to entertain any negative thoughts. Whatever he was enduring at that moment, he would get better. We instead would watch his favorite shows like *Breaking Bad* and the National Geographic channel. I was right there by his side, fighting for him, loving him, and comforting him—doing all in my power to make it bearable for my son.

The weeks that he did not have chemotherapy were spent doing the things that he loved. He spent time with his son, doing different activities like going skating, or going to the amusement park. It was important for him to be a good father to his child. He continued to enjoy the outdoors as much as he could: he would go to the beach or go fishing or hiking. He still loved cars but did not drive as much as before. He would go pick up food at his favorite restaurants or make other short trips. He enjoyed doing things with his family and love ones.

I watched my Buddy battle cancer for over two years. It was heart-wrenching. He went through so many changes, both physically and mentally. Things did not get better—they only worsened. I could not understand why his treatment wasn't working. I cried as I watched him try to cope, yet I never lost faith and I continued to believe that he would be healed.

All the experimental treatments that he did were not working. After every treatment, they would do a CT scan of his lungs. They found that some tissues were shrinking while some were getting larger. I could see the disappointment in my son's eyes every time he got the results, and it made me angry and frustrated. I would punch things and cry hysterically. I had prayed to God so many times. Why was my boy not getting better?

"Mom! Stop!" he would say. "You only make me miserable when you behave like this!"

I would stare at him and know he was right. Seeing me so upset was not doing him any good. He had enough to deal with. He was the one battling the cancer, after all. I just wanted my child to get better and get back to his life.

We decided to try some natural methods. My son had researched the topic and he drank special teas, shakes, and ate special foods. Sometimes he would say that he felt better, but there were no marked changes. There were a few times when he became frustrated, though he did not complain often.

At one point, he made plans to move out and make a life with his girlfriend. When he realized that this was not going to happen, he became angry and began to yell at me and say very mean things. He accused me of never allowing him to live his own life and of being too over-protective. He said he had never had the opportunity to be his own person.

My son had always been blunt when it came to what was on his mind, no matter how upsetting it might be to others. It was as if he was blaming me for his condition. His words made me cry. The only thing I was guilty of was living for my children.

Buddy never wanted anyone to feel sorry for him, nor did he want most people to know about his cancer. I remember the first time I told his friend, one of the homeless boys he had brought home years before. He was shocked to find out that my son had been so ill and that he had not been aware of it. At home, he did not want anyone to help him with anything. There were days when he was weak and tired, but he would still drive himself to the treatment center. I was not much help, as I could not drive. I worried about him getting into an accident. There were also times when I could not accompany him on his trips to the clinic. I would have to work or at times I had appointments of my own. I would suggest that he get someone else to drive him, and he was refuse and give me a hard time. –

"Mom, I do not want to ask anyone to take me anywhere or do anything for me," he would say angrily. "I don't wish to bother anyone. I just want you."

"Buddy," I replied, "I know how you feel, but I can't make it today. You know how much I wish I could be there, but sometimes I just can't." I would plead for his understanding, and finally he would agree to let a family member go with him. My husband took him many times as they had a good relationship.

My entire life revolved around my son and caring for him was my focus. I tried to make his life as comfortable and happy as possible, and I was grateful that I could be there to care for him. My life was full and extremely busy. I worked with the children in day care, but at every opportunity I would leave them in the care of another supervisor and go to him, even if it was just for a few minutes. I also continued to care for my family in the best way I could. I was thankful for my understanding husband, who was willing to work with me through this crisis.

I did not go out much and the few times I did it was only for a short period. I was tired, but it seemed I had always been tired, so I didn't let it get to me. I did not want to believe that my son was going to die and I continued to pray. I would tell my friends and family that he was getting better, though I could see the disbelief in their faces. Some of them expressed concern for my state of mind. He was concerned about my denial as well, and he tried to talk with me about it.

"I do not want to talk with you about dying, Buddy," I would say and immediately change the subject.

I tried to convince him that he would be okay, but he did not believe me. He was aware and accepting of what was happening to his body. He always accepted the reality of his cancer, though he wanted to live. He tried to get loved ones to talk with me, but I was unwilling. I chose not to believe that my son was going to die and leave me behind.

As his mother, believing that he was going to die meant that I was giving up on him. I could never, ever give up on my child and I was willing to fight and have faith until I died. This was my son, whom I loved more than life itself. I had prayed so many times, asking God to spare his life and take mine instead. I had lived my life, but he had just started his and had so much to live for. My son was everything to me and every day I showed him how much I loved him. I knew he was in turn grateful as I saw it in his big brown eyes every time he looked at me. One day, he ordered me a Pandora bracelet, which left me in tears. I told him he did not have to do that, but he insisted that I deserved it.

Buddy and I talked for long periods of time—about everything. He spoke to me in depth about my life and what I needed to do to be happy. He told me to focus on myself and not let people take advantage of me. He told me to not let people's actions surprise me so much and that I should expect little from others—especially love ones. I didn't understand at times why he said these sorts of things to me, but I was happy that he was telling me how he really felt. He wanted me to always be a part of his son's life and reminded me that I had rights as a grandmother. We talked about my difficult childhood and why it meant so much to me for him to be happy. My son wanted *me* to be happy and to do the things that I had dreamt of. I had only one wish: that he would get better and live a long, prosperous life.

Chapter 6

"Once a man, twice a child," is an old saying in my culture. I never understood what this meant until now. It means that one comes into this world as a baby and must be cared for until they can take care of themselves. They gain independence and build a life until they become old or sick and once again need assistance. This is what happened to my Buddy. His entire life changed, and he was totally dependent on me for everything once more, like the time when he was a baby. In time, he could no longer bathe himself or brush his teeth. I was not prepared for these devastating changes.

After three and a half years of battling cancer, it finally started to take its toll on my son's body. He was confined to a wheelchair since he was too weak to walk. He had lost a lot of weight and was very frail. He had to be on oxygen twenty-four hours a day as he could not breathe on his own. Portable oxygen devices were delivered to the house on a regular basis. I continued doing all I could to help him, from medical treatments to home remedies. He began to cough up blood, which terrified me. His doctors wanted to run more tests.

After the tests were completed, the doctors informed me that my son's cancer was worse. This was not the news I wanted to hear. They recommended that he be admitted to a hospital where he could be cared for by professionals who would see to his every comfort before he passed. My son did not want to go to a hospital. He only wanted me to care for him. Nurses had only come to our home to check his vital signs and monitor his care.

"Buddy," I said, "the doctors only want you to be comfortable since you are very sick. There are trained professionals who can give you everything you need." In truth, the doctor had told me that if my son did not receive hospice care, that he would die in a horrible and painful way. Still, I let him decide what he wanted to do.

"Ask the doctor how long I have, and then I will make a decision," he said.

I was quite taken back by his request, but immediately called his doctor. I left a message asking him to phone me as soon as possible. It was not easy caring for my sick son, who needed so much attention. I was physically and emotionally exhausted, but I took comfort in knowing that God had placed me there when my Buddy needed me most. I was glad that my job was in my home, so that I could run to him whenever he needed me.

When it came to any major decision concerning my son's overall wellbeing, I always gave him the power to decide for himself what he wanted. Although he was very sick, I did not want to take that away from him. He had lost so much to cancer and I did not want him to feel like he had no voice or that he was incompetent in any way. It had been difficult enough for him to accept the fact that he could no longer be as independent as he had been. He continued to educate himself about his cancer and constantly researched any new discoveries linked to ASPS. His sisters shared information with him at times as well. My son did not want to die: that I was sure about.

One day, he found a little hope while researching his cancer. He was excited to tell me about this German doctor who specialized in ASPS. The doctor had performed a few successful surgeries on patients. Some of the patients testified that he had saved their lives. My son was very excited and asked that I get in contact with this doctor. I immediately got in touch with his office and he requested that I sent my Buddy's CD and medical records so that he and his staff could take a look at them. I was also told the surgery would cost a hundred thousand dollars.

"Mom, where are we going to get all that money?" He asked me after I hung up the phone.

"Don't worry, Buddy," I replied. "I will find it." I saw the gleam of hope in his eyes, and I could not take that away from him. I smiled and said, "Have I ever let you down before?"

I spent the next few weeks trying to figure out how I was going to come up with the money. Could I get a loan? Could I refinance my home? I had no idea how I was going to make this happen, but I would get the money somehow. I refused to believe my son was going to die. Now that it seemed he had a chance, I had to do everything in my power. Images of my son getting better filled my mind as I looked at my accounts and assets and struggled to find a way.

Weeks later, I got a called from the German doctor's office who gave me disappointing news. He informed me that my son was not a candidate for the surgery. He believed that my son's cancer was too advanced and that there was nothing that could be done to help him. I was crushed, especially when I had to tell him the news. I watched as the hope drained from his eyes and I tried to comfort him.

"Don't worry, Buddy. You will be okay," I said as I hugged him. "Doctors are not always right."

"Mom, why can't you accept that I am going to die?" he asked me quietly.

"No, son, you will not die." I lay down next to him, holding his hand as he relaxed. I refused to believe the doctors, my family, and especially not my son. I had to have faith.

I looked at my son often with tears in my eyes. I would recall how strong and healthy he had been before the cancer. He had filled my life with excitement for his future. When I remembered how hyperactive he had been as a child, and yet now he had no energy to do anything, it broke my heart. Even feeding himself had become difficult. I prayed to God and asked him why. My grandson needed his father to teach him how to be a good man. They had many adventures yet in store.

I saw how his eyes lit up every time he saw his son. He was still a preschooler and the love they shared was obvious when they were together. When my son became too weak to play with his son, they would just lie together and cuddle.

Time wore on and my Buddy continued to get worse. He could no longer take medication and it had to be administered through his anus. He was losing his speech, but his other senses were still intact. He was still attentive and aware of his surroundings. The nurses had increased his meds from five to seven pills. I would put the seven pills in his hand and he would count and give me two back. When I told him to take the others, he became agitated and refused.

My son's primary doctor finally called me back after I had left a message. We spoke about his condition and I asked how long he had to live. "Three months or less" was his reply.

This was very difficult news to comprehend as his mother and I tried to deal with it the best I could. I tried to remain buoyant. I thought of when my son was first diagnosed, and how they had only given him a few months. Here is was, four years later. Doctors were not always right. I continued to hope for a miracle. No one, not the doctors nor family or friends could convince me otherwise. Since I saw him every day, I didn't see how much he had failed. Nurses gave me literature on preparing for death and I brushed them aside. How could I accept that my Buddy was going to die? That would be giving up on him, and that was out of the question. He begged me to prepare for his death on many occasions, but I would not consider it. I saw the deep concern in everyone's eyes as I continued on in my denial.

My son made his decision and soon started hospice care after I let him know what the doctor had said. He got the care he needed from doctors, nurses, home health aides, spiritual counselors and social workers. They took turns coming to our home as I continued to care for him as well. I knew him better than anyone: every sound, every movement, every facial expression meant something that only I could interpret. There were times when it was painful to look at my son, since he had changed so drastically. Remarkably, he still had all his senses. There were times when I spoke to him, and though he did not answer I knew he understood me. It took me back to the days when he was a baby and I talked to him about everything. I had seen the love in his eyes and it gave me the comfort I needed.

I would clean my Buddy's teeth and tongue, bathe him, feed him, and massage his thin, wracked body. In time, I had to put him in diapers. At first, he refused to pee in it and he tried to pull it off.

"Buddy, you can do whatever you want in this underwear," I said with a smile. I knew he was struggling with the idea of wetting himself. He was always so picky about his appearance.

"Mommy not mad?" he mumbled, looking at me with questioning eyes.

"No, Mommy not mad," I reassured him. "Mommy bought this beautiful underwear just for you. You can make whatever you want in them."

That was how I got him to use the diapers. He still fought me on many things, though he was tired. His body was losing the battle, but his mind stayed strong. I admired his will and his courage, and they motivated me as well.

"Mom," he said one day, "did you see that little girl dancing?"

"What little girl?" I asked as I looked about the bedroom.

"The little girl over there—she is dancing," he replied, looking across the room. "Don't you see her, Mom?"

"There is no one there, Buddy," I replied softly with a puzzled look.

"Yes, Mom, she is right there," he insisted.

I realized my son was hallucinating. The doctors said it might happen and that it was normal. There were others and he would tell me about them, all the while slurring his speech. He would see children dancing, and once he asked me if I saw the guy in the room. I would always tell him that no one was there. Once, he told me he saw Jesus walking. I was astonished at this as he was not a Christian. I had taken him to church and read him Bible stories when he was younger, but he was fascinated with science and evolution. He would give me an explanation for everything. Many argued with his beliefs, but he was not swayed. I was a strong believer in God, however, and when he called out Jesus' name I was both shocked and relieved. I believed that Jesus came into this world to die for the sins of mankind.

One of the things that my son wanted in his final days was to go outside, to feel the wind against his skin and the sun on his face. Being outside would give him peace and tranquility. I spoke to the doctor, but he told me that he should not go outside. His immune system was very low and he could easily get an infection. When I told my son what the doctor had said, he became very sad.

My Buddy was now in and out of a coma and his health was deteriorating with every passing day. Family members continued to spend time with him, talking to him or just lying next to him. His youngest sister would take her son to his room and place him on the bed, close to him. His son and his mother would also come by. Everyone was coping in their own way. He had been a huge part of their lives and it was hard for them to see him so sick and helpless. He was their big brother, their problem-solver, partner in crime and so much more.

One day, I was with my son in his room, caring for him like I always did. I was about to change the linens on his bed when the nurse asked me if she could do it instead.

"That's all right, I can do it," I said politely. I had been doing it for so long and did not have a problem continuing to do it.

She insisted and reluctantly I agreed and walked out of the room. I stood in the doorway, looking in. The image of a very sick, weak, helpless man who was all bones filled my mind and sent shockwaves through my brain as the nurse helped him to the bed. It was as though I was seeing this person for the very first time. This man was my son, my Buddy whom I loved more than life itself—and he was dying. I started to cry as reality hit me like a ton of bricks. How could I not have seen this? Why couldn't I have seen how sick he was? I started feeling guilty because I had told him over and over that he was going to be all right. I lied: I had lied to my son. How could I lie to my son? He was not going to get better. I saw that he was suffering, and I cried even more. At that moment, I prayed that God would take him. I did not want my Buddy to suffer anymore.

"My son is dying," I said. I began to sob as I walked up to the nurse. "My son is really dying."

"Thank God," the nurse replied, taking a deep breath as she looked at me.

"What do you mean 'Thank God'?" I asked in surprise. This was not what I expected to hear from a professional.

"I do not mean any disrespect, Ma'am," she replied calmly. "I am just thankful that you have finally accepted the fact that your son is dying. We were very worried about you."

I talked to the nurse and other workers about my Buddy for hours. I told them about his childhood up to that point: his most amazing moments, his likes, dislikes, milestones and everything I could think of about my son. They listened quietly as I went on about him with love and pride in my voice. There were moments filled with intense emotion and I would sob as they comforted me. Talking about him was therapeutic. I had accepted his fate and what was to come. –

After talking for a long time, I went to my son as he lay weak and comatose on his bed. I massaged his back, legs and hands and I kissed him. I lay beside him as my mind drifted. I loved him so much; I did not want him to go on this way, sick and suffering. I had fought for so long because I wanted him to be well again. I honestly believed that my faith and love would make him better, but I was wrong. It was never going to happen. My Buddy was dying and that was my reality. This was not the kind of life I wanted for him. Tears ran down my face as I comprehended my selfishness in wanting him to live under these circumstances. I lay there with my son in my arms and sobbed some more. The gift of death was what my Buddy needed now, and I prayed for it. I prayed hard that he would find peace.

Chapter 7

There are some moments in life that are quite unforgettable. Moments that, even if you try to forget, your heart and mind will not allow you to do so. These are moments that will stay with you forever. Some of them are great, like a marriage or the birth of a child—others are devastating. On February 20th, 2013, my son lost his battle with cancer. This is a day that I will never forget as long as I live. What happened on that day is still vivid in my memory.

It was a beautiful morning and the sun was shining brightly. There were already signs that it was going to be another hot day. It was extremely busy at my house, as it was to be inspected at some time that day. When you are a foster mother or a daycare owner, inspections are mandatory. The inspectors would come to my home and scrutinize everything, from safety to the children's menu. They wanted to make sure that the children were well cared for and that I was conforming to state regulations.

I had been working hard to get the place ready for several days. The preparations helped keep my mind off what was happening with my son. Every time I thought of a future without him, I began to cry. I tried to be strong and cherish every moment with him, but time was running out. As I looked over my house one last time, checking that all was in order, I asked my husband to go and see to him.

My husband returned shortly and told me that my son was making strange sounds. He had been in and out of a coma for the past few weeks. I immediately ran to him and did my usual routine, cleaning him and administering medication. He started making the sounds again and I phoned the nurse. She assured me that she would come by later to check on him. I lay down next to my son and touched his hands and forehead while I talked to him. He continued making sounds as if he wanted to talk to me. –

"What's wrong, Buddy?" I whispered as tears filled my eyes. "Do you want to talk to Mommy? You can talk to me."

When he made the sounds again, I could tell that he knew that I was there, talking to him.

"You are ready to go, right Buddy?" I murmured. I looked at his face and knew that he understood me. He had been fighting for so long and he was exhausted. "You can go now," I said.

I got up from his bed and went to the window and quickly pulled the curtains back, allowing the rays of sunlight to come in. The sun lit up the room, giving it a vibrant feeling. I knew I would make my son happy to feel the sun one last time.

"Baby, go. Fly away like a butterfly," I said as I looked into his face and held him in my arms. I cried, knowing it was time for me to let go. I then felt his frail hands touch my leg and he forcefully pulled his body into me, embracing me. He had not done this in a very long time. I knew at that moment he had heard me. The pulse Oximetry, a device that measures oxygen in the blood, began to beep loudly. I knew he had left me, but I was still in shock.

I started screaming loudly, calling out for my oldest son, who immediately rushed in. He looked at the pulse Oximetry for a few seconds before he confirmed that my Buddy was dead. He then helped me to take care of some basic things, because I could not function. I was broken and emotional. He phoned the other family members and the doctors at Research University. I was drowning in reality: my son was gone. My Buddy....

Soon the other children came home and they were crying hysterically. We cried and comforted one another, trying to deal with our loss. I had no idea how news of my son's death traveled through the community, but within an hour my house was crowded with friends and acquaintances that had come to offer condolences. I tried my best to hold it together.

A short time later, the staff from the University arrived to take his body away. I was not ready. My son had arranged to give his body over for research at a leading private research university. When he had first told me about it, I was shocked and could not understand why he wanted to do that. He explained to me that there was lots of research that needed to be done for his form of cancer, and that he wanted to provide data that might find a cure and save lives. My son had the biggest heart, and I respected him even more for this decision.

"Can I have a few more minutes with my son?" I asked when the men from the University arrived. Everything was happening so fast. I felt helpless and weak. My eldest son convinced them to give me a little more time. They agreed to two more hours. I was told that after they had done what they needed I could have the body back for a funeral service and burial. I did not waste any time pondering on that because I knew that was something that my son hadn't wanted: he did not want to be seen and remembered by his loved ones with parts of his body missing or in disarray.

I sat there with my son's cold, lifeless body as sobbing people continued to pay their last respects. It was a very emotional and painful time for everyone. My son who had been a huge part of our lives was no more. I cried and cried as I thought about living my life without him. I watched as they finally came and took him away, knowing my life would never be the same. And it wasn't....

The days turned into weeks and the weeks into months as my life changed for the worse and I mourned the death of my son. A huge part of my heart had been ripped from me. He was part of my existence. I had built my entire life around him and my family, and now he was gone. I was not myself. I could not eat or sleep and I was consumed with thoughts of only him. There were moments when I pictured him walking in the door, or doing some of the fun things he used to do. Every part of the house reminded me of him. I left his room just the way he had left it and let no one touch a thing. I would sit alone and sob as I remembered all the fun things we used to do. We used to sit together outside in our backyard, but I could not bring myself to do it now that he was gone. I cried myself to sleep at night, thinking about him all the time. I entered into serious depression and withdrew from everyone around me.

Friends and loved ones tried to comfort me and be there for me, but I pushed them away. I felt as though they wanted me to act in a certain sort of way, but I could not. They constantly told me things would get better. How was that possible? I honestly believed no one understood what I was going through or how I felt. I needed an escape: I was suffocating and the walls were closing in on me. I turned to smoking and drinking heavily to deal with the pain. They only provided temporary relief. The moments when I was sober I mentally fought for my sanity. I began to blame myself and was guilt-ridden over the way I had handled my son's diagnosis. Why did I lie to my son about his condition? He was dying and for years I tried to persuade him that he wasn't. What kind of a mother would do that to her child? I became angry with myself.

"Was I a good mother?" I asked myself constantly. I believed that I was not. I should have told my son the truth about his sickness. I had always encouraged my children to be honest, and now I was the biggest hypocrite. I was a walking zombie, unable to care for myself, let alone my family. I continued to push people away. I believed I was unattractive and worthless, and that my family was better off without me. I had spent my entire life caring for others, and now I did not want to be bothered. I was in my own personal hell, and no one could reach me.

My mother, concerned over my health and well-being, visited from my homeland. She was instrumental in making me see that I could not go on living the way I was. She talked with me and she listened as I would break down, pouring out my grief. I needed a mother's love and she gave it to me especially when I needed it the most, never judging me. We had never had that kind of relationship in the past, and it was a great comfort to me. That was the beginning of my healing process.

I decided to pull myself out of the dark hole that had become my life. I stopped smoking and ceased other unhealthy behaviors. It was not easy, but I persevered. I thought of the kind of life that my son had wanted me to live, and I began to live it. I began keeping a journal, meditating and praying regularly. Gradually, I began to be myself again. I resolved to take control of my life and, besides loving others, love myself.

I often reflected on all the horrible things I had been through in my life, things that could have broken me, but didn't: poverty, my father's death, rape and molestation, a horrible first marriage, and fighting cancer myself. I had never stopped fighting through all of it. All those experiences had not changed me into a bitter person. They only made me stronger. I learned to tap into my inner strength and keep moving forward. If I continued on my former path, I was no good to anyone, and I had children who still needed their mother, as well as a patient husband who loved me.

I struggled to become stronger, but mentally I was tempted to fall back into unhealthy behaviors. This would happen when I was reminded of my son in some way. There were major family issues, unexpected events that tested my strength as well. My heart was battered once more and I wondered if I would ever have peace, if I would ever be happy again. What was I doing wrong? Was I a good person?

I was consumed with self-doubt until I would think of my Buddy's words. I "should not be surprised by anyone's actions—especially my love ones". It was as if my boy had seen into the future. His words gave me comfort. My son believed in my strength and forgave my weaknesses. He loved me unconditionally.

As time went by, I did many things to help keep my son's memory alive. I wanted everyone to know how special he was. When I did those things, it made me so much happier. I opened a GoFundMe account in his name in order to help raise funds for research. The money collected was given to the hospital where my son was treated, to assist in researching ASPS. Many young people were diagnosed with the condition that took his life. I helped organize a walk in his memory. Friends and family wore t-shirts and wristbands with his name and cause written on them. Doing these things helped me and there was so much more I wanted to do. I felt close to him when I organized these events. I imagined all sorts of other benefits like car washes and hikes, but I could not do it alone and could not get enough support. Sadly, I had to close his foundation.

Chapter 8

It has been five years since I lost my sweet child. There are so many things that still remind me of him and the love that we shared. Sometimes I find myself thinking about a happy moment that we had together and I smile. Other times, I miss him like crazy and wish he were here with me. Every year, on the anniversary of his death, I do something special. This year I took his son, youngest brother and cousins to see the movie *Peter Rabbit*. I recalled the way my Buddy had loved the character and I smiled.

I do not cry anymore for losing my son. I honestly believe that he is in a better place—a place where he is not suffering anymore. He was Mommy's boy as a baby, was very adventurous and had a troublesome start in life. Then, he became calmer and figured out what was most important. He fell in love, but he also knew hurt and disappointment. He became a father, the highlight of his life. My son lived a full life though he died young. I look at his child sometimes and am very thankful that my son left me this little miracle. He reminds me of his father often with the little things he does. I also see how his death affected my family and how they have struggled to go on without him. It is especially not easy for his younger sister. She posts pictures, quotes, and other memories of him on her social media pages. It is her way of keeping her big brother alive.

My Buddy will forever stay alive in my heart. This is something that no one, not even time can take away from me. We had a great love and a rare bond. I honestly believe that he was the best part of me. He was with me through the dark times, and he was my inspiration and my motivator. I became a stronger person because of his faith in me. He helped me conquer my fears and changed my life for the better.

I continued doing simple things to make sure that he was still present in my life and that his memory lived on. I built him a beautiful headstone. I went to the beach that he loved so much and collected the stone, which I carved myself with hands of love. On it, I wrote "Buddy, the world has lost a light in you, but you have gained a star in heaven." I planted a flower garden in my yard and placed the stone in it. It is a tribute to his love for nature and the great outdoors. Every time I look at the beautiful flowers, I think of him.

What doesn't break you surely makes you stronger. When I think back on how broken and devastated I was when I lost my son and how far I have since come, I am thankful. I talk to God daily about all the things I have been through, and I know that, because of my faith in him, I am now doing much better. I have been through so many difficult and painful moments and I am still standing strong. Those hardships could have made anyone lose their sanity, but I did not. God has-been with me every step of the way and I am thankful. I did not always think this, but I am learning to accept things as they are. Now, as I think about my son, I am appreciative for the miracle that God gave to me. When my Buddy was diagnosed, he was given only months to live. I had him for almost four years, which was truly miraculous. God only took him when I was capable of accepting his destiny, and he was happy to let go because I believed. I will never forget how peaceful he was when he drew his last breath.

When my son died, I remember thinking "Why him?" He was not perfect, but he was an amazing human being. Why couldn't it have been me? Was there something else I could have done? These are questions I no longer ask myself. Everything in my life has happened for a reason, even the horrible things. I take my life a day at a time. I know I did the best I could for my son.

I am at the point in my life where I do not take anything or anyone for granted. Every day I work to be the best person I can be. I try to no longer worry about the things I cannot change. People will always disappoint, and I am learning not to let it get to me. I focus on myself more, as my son suggested that I do. I eat healthy and take long walks. I take vacations. I am a stronger, better me.

There are many things that I am thankful for in my life. I have a loving husband who had stood by my side through good and bad times. My son's only child is a part of my life and I have him near me. I have a younger son who is a burst of energy like his older brother, and my other children and grandchildren put a smile on my face whenever I see them. I now focus on the important things in life. I now choose to celebrate my child, instead of mourning him. I will celebrate him as long as I live. I know that he is looking down on me and I hold on to the belief that I will see him again. My Buddy was not perfect, but he was perfect to me.

My son's, body was cremated and I now have the ashes in my possession. The doctors at the university, where he had given his body for research, had a small ceremony for families and loved ones. They expressed their gratitude and I felt proud that my Buddy was part of such an important cause. They gave me his ashes, the only physical part of him that remains. I cannot part with them, though friends and family suggest that I should let them fly off into the ocean or in some other location. I am not mentally prepared to let him go entirely. I believe there will come a time when I will know what to do. It will be my choice. Until then, my Buddy remains with me.

Lastly, God has placed a wonderful woman in my life. The fact that she has written my story is truly a miracle. Writing this book was very therapeutic for me. Thanks, Sal.

Chapter 9

From the moment my son was diagnosed with cancer up until the time he passed away, there were friends and loved ones who were there. They offered their love and support which I am very grateful for. Many had been there throughout his life and contributed to the type of person he was. I have saved some of their letters and written testimonies that I look at from time to time. My son was loved and admired by many and I know that he is greatly missed. I believe that he had left behind lasting impressions which would forever be remembered by the people whose life he had touched. This book is dedicated to everyone who was part of my Buddy's life. Thank you for being there and sharing moments with him.

I have written letters in my journal while I took care of my sick son and after his passing. There were so many emotions that I was dealing with at that time. Sometimes writing them gave me the opportunity to say how I really feel – without being judged by anyone. Here are some letters and notes that I have written to my Buddy.

10TH October 2010

As the days pass and we are given results and try to come to teams with the situation at hand, we must show strength. We are not going to give up; we will fight everyday together – as a family. The test that the lord has put before us is not aimed towards one person. It is not Buddy alone being tested, it's all of us.

'We walk by faith but not and not by sight.'

(Here we go)

10.15.2010

Dear Buddy I am praying that you get better soon. It does not matter what the doctor said, I know that you will get better. Mom

10.19. 2010

My Dearest son,

Today I built up the nerve to write in this book. The day I found out that you had cancer was the hardest day of my life. It's beyond belief since my kids are my life. I have put all of my life and my dreams in my children and now I have to face something that is so hard. That is the beginning of our lives since we have to fight the fight of our life - The hardest fight of our lifetime. God have given me the faith and strength to fight this fight with you. Baby I love you more than life itself and could not imagine life without you. God is just testing our love and faith thus making us a better family. Don't ever give up my son, keep on fighting. Keep on living and keep God's love. You are my son now and forever.

Love your Mom

July 13th 2011 12:17am

The Rainbow car

'When we were little, driving on the freeway,

We would fantasize about what the car in the front of all the other cars would be like.

You, my sister and I agreed it was a car that reflected every color of the rainbow.

Now that I am older, I know the truth. There was no rainbow car leading all the other cars. That was us being kids, believing in magic, dancing to every fairy tale beat...' Kita

After my Buddy died

May 27.2014

Dear Buddy,

It's mom. I just meet a roadblock. It's something that I can't solve. I knew if you were here you would have given me your advice and we would have talked about it. I miss you so much. It is so hard for me to accept that you are not here.

I know that everything that I have been through in my life, had led me to this one single moment in my life.

I never thought that you were going to die and this was my greatest flaw. I hope Buddy; you know how much I love you. I love you more than everything in this life and beyond.

I know that my life would never be the same. Your life has changed mine forever. I never thought that it was possible to love someone the way that I love you buddy. Please help me to understand why I came into this life. It seems that everything was bad from the very start.

Every day I live it gets harder. I am so afraid to count on the good and positive things. Nothing seems to be for me. Today I feel like my life is not worth living. You were my everything - a big part of me has left with you. I do not know if I would get it back. I love all my children. There is so much now that I understand about myself because of you. I love you for that. You were a great son. It's so sad that you will not get to meet your sister kita's baby. Love Mom

June 14. 2014

Dear Buddy,

Today is very sad for me. There are so many things that I am dealing with right now. I am thinking about your son little Jordan. This is his first father's day without you.

I am feeling helpless without you. I can't believe how much things that we talked about. I talked to you about so many different things. What a great love we shared.

I need you so much in my life. They say that time will heal all wounds but mines never will. I just want you back badly. I want you back! I want you back! My heart will never heal. It is broken.

I also finish my Pandora bracelet and it's beautiful. Thank you.

I love you more.

Mom

Feb 12. 2016

Dear Buddy,

Today is two years you have passed away. I was very sad and broken and still can't believe that you are not here. I am going crazy since you are not here. I believe in God and know that you are in a better place, waiting for me. Mom

The day that you passed away – everything went away. I can't even explain. The whole family went crazy and lost their mind.

Without you I can hear a pin drop. My days are just so long and I am lost in the dark and can't find my way out. Please help me find my way out.

Love you forever. Mom

Presently

I have been a very important part of Buddy's life. I was very pleased to see his transition into the wonderful young man that he became, after all of life's challenges as a teenager growing up. I know that have he been alive today, things would have been better in many ways for everyone – especially his family.

'When I was a little girl, I made some waffles and took them into the dining room to eat. You asked me if you could cut them for me. You cut them into four big pieces and then you ate them. I never got upset. I would have given you anything and done anything to see you happy. I love you so intensely and I always felt so complete when I was the cause of your happiness. I miss you and I love you.'

Dear Buddy,

Your son misses you. My heart breaks for him especially when it's his birthday, father's day or special holidays that you two should be spending together as a family. We wish that you were here.

Love mom

My Buddy,

I miss you so very much. A few weeks ago your son's mother showed me pictures and I could not stop crying as I looked at them. They were pictures of you, your son and his mom which I have never seen before. There were so much love and promise in those pictures. I cried for that loss - no one understood why I was reacting in this manner since you have died years ago. I miss you so much. All though I have accepted the reality that you are not here with me physically, I will never stop missing you.

Mom

Chapter 10

'A picture is worth ten thousand words,'
Fred R Barnard.

Some people say that looking at a picture can tell you a million things. This is very true for me. I look at pictures of my wonderful son that was taken throughout his life and they remind me of so many moments. Sometimes I smile, and other times I burst into tears. These photos are very special to me. They are also the only reminders that his son has of his father. Though his memory lives in my heart, I am grateful for these photos. I can look at his handsome face and remember my Buddy. I wish that I can share them with you so that you can see how special he was to me and the people who he loved. These pictures show the different stages of his life - some with the people who have touched his life in a special way. My Buddy may have passed away but I know that he is with me every day. I may not be able to see or hear him but I know that he is always near. He was a beautiful soul and perfect to me. I would never forget him since he had left lasting prints in my life. Remembering him is so easy because I do it every day but missing him is a heartache that will never go away. The memories of him I hold in my heart forever until we meet again.